Your Amazing Itty Bitty™ Diabetes Book

15 Key Steps to Understanding, Managing and Living a Full Life with Diabetes

Himmet Dajee, MD, FACS

Published by Itty Bitty™ Publishing
A subsidiary of S & P Productions, Inc.

Printed in the United States of America

Itty Bitty Publishing
311 Main Street, Suite D0
El Segundo, CA 90245
(310) 640-8885

ISBN: 978-1-7329566-7-4

The author assumes no responsibility or liability for any errors or omissions in the content of this book. The topic of discussion is not a substitute for professional medical advice, diagnosis, or treatment. The medical disclaimer specifies that the information provided is for informational or educational purposes only and does not constitute professional advice.

This information is not intended to replace a consultation with an appropriately qualified medical practitioner.

Dedication

This book is dedicated to my wife and daughters who have always been vigilant in assuring that I control my blood glucose and predicted when it was on the verge of being abnormal.

Your family needs to be aware of the early signs and symptoms of abnormal blood glucose levels. By doing so they can assist in preventing adverse events by intervening in a timely fashion. Sharing your diagnosis with family and friends may be key in preventing a catastrophic event from happening.

Stop by our Itty Bitty™ website to find
interesting blog entries regarding Diabetes

www.IttyBittyPublishing.com

Or contact Himmet Dajee, MD, FACS at

hdajeemd@aol.com

Table of Contents

Introduction

At all costs, you want to avoid becoming a diabetic. Do not be secretive about your diagnosis as many people have friends and family who are compassionate and willing to help you in times of crisis. You can live a normal productive life, and I am living proof of that. As a 49-year-old cardiac surgeon, I had my chest opened for coronary bypass surgery. Subsequently, I took all the advice about medication, exercise, and lowering stress to a minimum. I returned to my practice six weeks later.

Later, I married and started a family. Fifteen years later I had to have another surgery, but this time I retired from practice and my goal was to spend time with my wife and daughters. Not satisfied with being idle, six months later I became Medical Director at a managed health plan. Sixteen years later I am still active with the plan. During this time, I wrote my memoir.

My advice to you:

1. Avoid being alone. Loneliness is a risk factor for coronary artery disease.
2. Do not deny you are diabetic; you cannot live in a shadow.
3. Your physician and diabetic educator are there to assist you.
4. Avoid undue stress in life; meditation helps.

Step 1
The Epidemic of Diabetes

Diabetes is a worldwide epidemic; no one is immune to it. Initially, it was considered a disease of wealthy nations, but as living standards improved in India, China, Africa and other poorer countries, the rest of the world was introduced to fast food. The incidence of diabetes followed with devastating health outcomes.

The following are some of the statistics you need to be aware of.

1. The number of people diagnosed with diabetes has doubled in 20 years.
2. About 35 million adults in the US have diabetes.
3. Diabetes is ranked as the seventh leading cause of death.
4. The effect of diabetes, unfortunately, ravages every organ in your body.
5. If you are at risk, get an eight-hour fasting blood glucose test every three years. If you are diagnosed as prediabetic then you must have blood tests yearly.

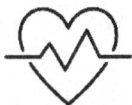

More About Diabetes

Over 84 million people are considered pre-diabetic. Many may be unaware they have had this silent condition for 8 to 10 years *before* diagnosis, but you don't have to be taken by surprise.

Other things you should know about diabetes:

- Diabetes is a disorder of insulin that is produced by specialized (beta) cells in the pancreas.
- If you have this illness, glucose uptake by your body tissue is impaired and cannot be used as an energy source.
- Thus, your blood glucose remains elevated, and the excess is eliminated in your urine along with water; therefore, you feel thirsty most of the time.
- Because energy or glucose is being lost you lose weight and remain fatigued and hungry.
- Diabetes is characterized as "starvation amid plenty."

Step 2
Classifications of Diabetes

There are three specific types of diabetes: Type 1, Type 2, and gestational. It is important for you as a diabetic to know the differences between each one and how they are treated.

1. Type 1 is more prevalent in children and young adults but can occur at any age. The beta cells of the pancreas are destroyed by autoimmunity; thus, no insulin is produced, and you have to self-inject insulin to keep blood glucose levels within normal range.
2. Type 2 is the most common type of diabetes (90-95%) in adults. Your body does not make insulin or does not use insulin well. It can develop at any age but occurs most frequently in middle age and older patients.
3. Gestational diabetes occurs in women who are pregnant. As a woman, you do not produce enough insulin to overcome insulin resistance, but potentially you are at risk of developing Type 2 diabetes later in life.

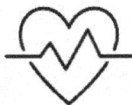

Other Causes of Diabetes

Aside from the three main types of diabetes, there are a significant number of other circumstances that can lead to this condition as well.

- Cystic fibrosis causes pancreatic scarring that impairs the beta cells that produce insulin.
- Pancreatitis and pancreatic cancer similarly impair the cells that produce insulin.
- Cushing's syndrome with increased cortisol levels and stress hormones.
- Acromegaly causes high growth hormone levels.
- Hemochromatosis builds up iron toxicity that kills the beta cells in the pancreas.
- You may develop diabetes if you have been prescribed niacin, diuretics, psychotropics, and HIV medications. In addition, antirejection and antiseizure medications, along with steroids for the treatment of colitis, lupus, asthma, and rheumatoid arthritis can also be attributed to diabetes.

This is a good time to talk to your doctor to check your blood glucose to see if you have any of the above disorders. We will come to a test later, called hemoglobin A1C which averages blood sugar levels over the past three months.

Step 3
Common Symptoms and Non-Insulin Treatments of Diabetes

This step covers the symptoms of diabetes to look for along with non-insulin treatments.
Unfortunately, at times there are no symptoms of diabetes. This is true in the prediabetic phase. It is initially a silent disease, but there can be ongoing damage that may fester for up to 10 years.

Some common warning signs to look for include:

1. Thirst
2. Dry mouth
3. Increased urination
4. Fatigue
5. Hunger
6. Dry itchy skin
7. Weight loss
8. Changes in vision
9. Paresthesia and numbness of feet and fingers
10. Recurrent infections
11. Delayed wound healing
12. Dark patches (acanthosis nigricans) on your skin including under the breast, armpits, and skin creases particularly in obese patients

See your doctor annually for a checkup if you think you are at risk or have family members who have diabetes.

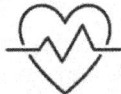

Non-Insulin Treatments for Diabetes

There have been many breakthroughs in the treatment of Type 2 diabetes. Two common types of treatment include oral medications and bariatric weight loss surgery.

- Ozempic is a once-a-week medication for Type 2 diabetes taken with or without food. Weight loss is a possibility.
- Trulicity is also a once-a-week medication for Type 2 diabetes taken with or without food. Men with (or who have had) medullary thyroid cancer or multiple endocrine neoplasias should not use this medication.
- Exenatide (bydureon) is a once-a-week medication.
- Victoza is a once-a-day medication.
- Weight loss surgery results in remission of diabetes by enforced food restriction, increased insulin sensitivity, and secretion. At least 60% of patients controlled their diabetes along with their BP. Triglycerides and cholesterol levels were lowered. Candidates for bariatric surgery need a body mass index (BMI) of above 30, having failed a physician-supervised weight loss program.

Additional Non-Insulin Treatments Include:

- Transplants
- Genetic Engineering

Step 4
Diagnostic Tests

Without proper testing, you could be risking your health as complications may occur without your knowledge. Eliminate the guesswork by seeing your doctor to have these important tests done.

Common blood tests include:

1. Fasting blood glucose, which requires eight hours of fasting before blood is drawn.
2. Random blood glucose: no fasting needed, test when symptoms are suspected.
3. HbA1c: No fasting needed, the test determines average blood glucose over the past three months. Not accurate in patients with anemia, sickle cell disease or pregnancy where there is a rapid turnover of hemoglobin.
   a. Frequency of testing is two times per year, or every three months when not meeting goals.
   b. Studies show that only 50% of diabetics reach their HbA1c levels.
   c. You are considered poorly controlled if HbA1c is > 9.3%.
   d. The range for good control is 6.5- 7.2%.

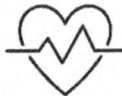

More About Testing for Diabetes

The following are additional types of blood tests to be aware of.

- Autoantibody testing looks for antibodies produced against insulin. This finding is common in Type 1 diabetes.
- In pregnancy, test for blood glucose levels no later than 12 weeks after birth to determine if the patient is a type II diabetic.

	HbA1c	Fasting B/G
Normal	<5.7	99 or <
Pre DM	5.7-6.4.	100-125
Diabetes	6.5 or >	126 or >

Urine Tests

Albumin and microalbumin (more sensitive) are early indicators of diabetic nephropathy.

Other Tests

Fasting lipids, total cholesterol, LDL, HDL, triglycerides, liver function tests, serum creatinine, and GFR for renal function are tests to be considered.

Step 5
Predisposition to Diabetes

There are several predispositions for diabetes. Some include ethnicity and genetics. You cannot choose your parents, so based on your DNA you may be at nonmodifiable risk for diabetes.

1. Ethnicity: Some nationalities are more at risk than others, including Latinos, African Americans, Alaskans, Native Americans, Asian Americans, and Pacific Islanders.
2. Genetics: Genes account for up to 65% of Type 1 diabetes. Type 2 has a higher familial risk, but only 10% of genes contribute to the illness.

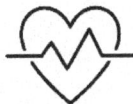

More About Predisposition to Diabetes

Socioeconomic factors play a significant role in
the exacerbation of diabetes. With fewer parks
and playgrounds, along with economic disparity,
you may find you are less active, making food
choices that are not in your best interest. This can
result in the following:

- Obesity or excess fat. A BMI of >30 is
  considered obese.
- A sedentary lifestyle that contributes to
  diabetes.
- Sleep deprivation can be harmful. Aim
  for 7-9 hours of sleep per night.
- Sleep apnea should be under control.
- Chronic stress contributes to illness.
- Age over 45 years is a risk factor for
  diabetes.
- Poor dietary habits work against you.
  Avoid fast and processed foods, sodas,
  foods high in fat and low in fiber, and
  alcohol. When shopping, always read
  food labels for sugar, salt, and fat content
  (the lower the better).

Step 6
Complications of Acute Diabetes

Complications and adverse outcomes from diabetes can be acute or chronic. In this step, we will be discussing acute diabetes.

Acute complications such as uncontrolled high glucose or low blood glucose can happen quickly and be life-threatening. Make sure your family members and friends are aware of these potential problems so they can initiate treatment or seek immediate help.

1. If you have signs of any of these complications, seek immediate medical treatment. Urgent attention may be needed to prevent life-threatening conditions.
2. Ketoacidosis (DKA) patients may have rapid breathing, nausea, vomiting, a central nervous malfunction with coma, and potential death.

Listen to your body for warning signs. Complications may take years of uncontrolled blood glucose levels to appear but can ultimately affect virtually every organ in your body.

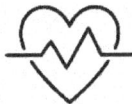

More About Acute Diabetes.

- Blood glucose does not enter your cells. Instead, the body uses fats for energy, and the term for the breakdown of these products is *ketones,* which are toxic when they accumulate.
- DKA is more prevalent in lower socio-economic individuals, along with those who can't afford or must discontinue insulin. People with a high rate of infections and drug users are also at risk for DKA.
- Hyperosmolar hyperglycemic syndrome and nonketotic coma are more common in Type 1 diabetics. With this serious condition, your glucose would be > 1000mg/dL without acidosis.
- Hypoglycemia is a serious condition that can be related to the medications you take. Excess insulin, oral medications, and a combination of inadequate food intake can lower your blood glucose, to < 70mg/dl.
- This may result in sweating, trembling, increased heart rate, irritability, dizziness, confusion, and unconsciousness with devastating outcomes.

Step 7
Chronic Complications

When possible, avoid persistent elevation of your blood glucose. Increased blood glucose levels over time can have severe and damaging effects on your blood vessels. Both small vessels (microvascular disease) and large vessels (macrovascular disease) are affected. In this step we will discuss microvascular disease.

Microvascular complications:

1. Eyes: *Retinopathy* affects the retina of your eye and can result in loss of vision.
   a. Results in 10,000 cases of blindness yearly in the US.
   b. Formation of weak retinal blood vessels causing hemorrhage.
   c. Retinal detachment from hemorrhages may occur.
2. Kidneys: *Nephropathy,* is a leading cause of kidney failure in the US. Albumin in the urine affects up to 7% of diabetic patients.
   a. Low-grade protein loss, initially (microalbuminuria) 30-299 mg/24 hour.
   b. If unattended, >500mg/24-hour loss is diabetic nephropathy.

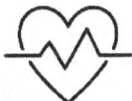

More About Chronic Diabetes

Neuropathy can also occur with prolonged elevation of blood sugar over an extended number of years. Symptoms may include:

- Numbness, tingling, and static electric charge-like pain.
- Lack of sensation resulting in an inability to feel a vibration, light touch, and temperature changes.
- Breakdown of skin with ulcerations and infection leading to gangrene of the feet.

Autonomic neuropathy damages nerves in the stomach and bowel. This may result in paralysis of the motility of the stomach with nausea, vomiting, constipation, or diarrhea.

- Inability to sweat
- Bladder abnormality
- Erectile dysfunction

Cardiac autonomic neuropathy complications include:

- Orthostatic hypotension, a drop of > 30 mm Hg systolic blood pressure and a drop of > 10 mm Hg in diastolic BP.
- Blunted heart rate response to exercise results in an insufficient rise in heart rate after exercise. Heart rate is slow to recover; this is predictive of cardio-vascular disease, causing mortality.

Step 8
Macrovascular Complications and Other Chronic Diseases

In people with diabetes, 68% of deaths happen because of heart and blood vessel problems. However, this can be prevented. In the next step we will discuss measures you can take to lessen your risk of developing diabetes.

The main problem with macrovascular disease is that a condition called atherosclerosis develops, which makes it harder for blood to flow through the large arteries. This happens because of ongoing swelling and buildup of fats on the artery walls, creating plaque which can rupture.

Macrovascular complications can have long-term effects on the body that include:

1. Coronary heart disease, heart failure or sudden death
2. Minor or Major stroke
3. Pains in the lower limbs (Claudication)
4. Arrhythmia – Irregular heart rhythm

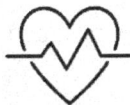

More About Chronic Diseases and Their Effect on Diabetes

As macrovascular disease progresses you may become at risk for any of the following:

- Coronaries: can lead to chest pain, heart attacks, or silent heart attacks, which are frequent in diabetics.
- Carotid: Carotid arteries in your neck can cause a small stroke or a temporary ischemic attack (TIA). These usually don't leave lasting damage or paralysis but might lead to some ongoing other problems, several months later.
- Cerebral: Arteries in the brain, that can get blocked due to atherosclerosis. This may cause cells in the brain to die because they don't get enough oxygen, leading to different levels of paralysis.

Peripheral Vascular Disease (PVD)

PVD happens when the arteries in your legs have atherosclerosis. This can cause low blood flow and might even lead to blockages. Pain in your calves, when you walk, may happen. If it's not treated, it could cause serious problems like gangrene, where muscles start to die, and may lead to amputation.

See your doctor annually for a checkup if you are at risk or have family members who have diabetes.

Step 9
Prevention of Diabetes

It can take a village to motivate changes to achieve good health when the alternatives could ruin your life. Seek support from family members, primary care physicians, pharmacists, nurses, nutritionists, and diabetic health educators.

1. Avoid a sedentary lifestyle! Be physically active for 30 minutes/day or 150 minutes/week. Examples: brisk walking, running, cycling, swimming, resistance exercises, and yoga.
2. Weight loss is imperative in prediabetes. You should lose 7-10% of your body weight, to prevent the progression of the disease.
3. Avoid excess starches and sugars, processsed foods with high fructose corn syrup, and fruit juices.
4. Consider vegetables like broccoli, cauliflower, and leafy greens. Your fruit options can include tomatoes, apples, and berries.
5. Fiber helps delay the absorption of sugars from the gut. Some high-fiber, protein, and vitamin-enriched options are beans, legumes, chickpeas, and lentils. A Mediterranean diet is low in fats and calories.

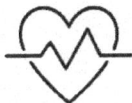

More About How Your Diet Can Help

Managing the size of your meals is important, as large meals may increase blood sugar levels. Eating smaller portions over several hours during the day can help you attain balanced levels, and smaller plates can help prevent overeating.

- Beneficial fats in your diet include unsaturated and polyunsaturated fats such as olive oil, sunflower and canola oils, and nuts such as almonds, flaxseed, walnuts, and pumpkin seeds. Fish: cod, salmon, sardines, mackerel, anchovies, tuna, and herring are also beneficial.
- Limit red meats.
- Smoking reduces oxygen in tissues and can result in insulin resistance. Consider taking smoking cessation classes to stop smoking.
- Control blood pressure and always consult your doctor if your blood pressure is high.
- Avoid stressful situations when possible. Elevated stress hormones such as cortisol increase the risk of high blood pressure, heart disease, and diabetes.

Step 10
Medication and Treatments

There are two primary treatment objectives. They are non-medical treatments that include diet and exercise and the use of prescription medications.

You will want to reduce blood glucose levels to a normal range to prevent morbidity and mortality.

1. Diet with calorie restrictions to limit carbohydrates and fats, while maintaining adequate proteins.
2. Exercise to move glucose into cells, so it does not elevate blood sugar.

You can also use medications to control diabetes.

1. French lilac was used as a folk remedy for diabetes during medieval times.
2. Synthalin, a guanidine byproduct from plants, was used briefly in the 1920s, but liver toxicity ceased its use.
3. Metformin, another biguanide, appeared in 1959. It was approved for use in the US in the 1990s.

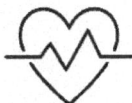

More About Medication and Treatment

- Sulfonylureas stimulate the release of insulin from beta cells in the pancreas.
- Biguanides decrease the production of glucose in the liver and increase the action of insulin on muscle and fat tissues.
- Thiazolidinedione reduces insulin resistance in muscles, the liver, and fat cells, and facilitates entry of glucose into those cells.
- Alpha-glucosidase inhibitors lower blood glucose by delaying the breakdown of carbohydrates and decreasing glucose absorption in the small bowel.
- Meglitinide (incretin mimetics) increases the release of insulin, decreases the release of glucose from the liver after a meal, and delays food emptying from the stomach.
- DPP-4 inhibitors release more insulin from the pancreas after meals and decrease the release of glucose from the liver.
- SGLT2 inhibitors act on the kidneys to remove glucose.

Most patients prefer oral medications because of their ease of use. However, when blood glucose remains elevated, alternative treatment is warranted. Welcome to insulin.

Step 11
Treatments and Injectables (Insulins and Non-insulins)

Before the discovery of insulin in 1921 by Frederick Banting and his assistant Charles Best (under the directorship of John Macleod from the University of Toronto), patients usually died within one to two years of the onset of diabetes.

1. There are rapid-acting insulins you inject 15 minutes before each meal, which peak in action at one hour and last two to four hours.
2. There are also short-acting insulins that reach the bloodstream within 30 minutes of injection. This type peaks in effect in two to three hours and lasts three to six hours.
3. Finally, there are intermediate-acting insulins that reach the bloodstream in two to four hours. They peak at four to 12 hours and work up to 18 hours.

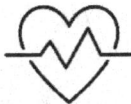

Treatments and Injectables Continued

Long-acting insulins keep your blood glucose stable the whole day and can last up to 18 hours.

- Insulins are taken by syringe or insulin pens and are administered with a needle injected under the skin. Insulin pumps are also available to deliver insulin periodically.
- Insulin pumps are approximately the size of a smartphone and are worn around the waist. The pumps are connected via a thin tube that is placed with a cannula under your belly skin. Acting like an artificial pancreas, pumps are a closed-loop insulin delivery system that monitors and checks blood glucose levels every five minutes. The pump then delivers an insulin dose as needed.
- Continuous glucose monitoring with a portable reader and sensor attached to the skin sends the tissue levels of glucose to the reader continuously for 14 days. This avoids multiple finger pricks to check blood glucose levels.

My advice during travel is to never run out of insulin. Scheduling your insulin dosing with your doctor is recommended since adjustments are needed for time zones and air travel. You always want to have enough insulin while traveling. Never pack insulin in your checked luggage. Be sure to carry it onboard with you.

Step 12
The Potential Financial Burden of Diabetes

The staggering and escalating costs of diabetes have ruined many families. Those who feel they cannot bear these exorbitant expenditures need a serious and urgent discussion with their physician, congressman, or senator.

Below are the economics of diabetes and the financial burden on our society.

1. The total cost of diabetes in the US as of 2017 is $327 billion.
2. Of that $327 billion, $237 billion is spent on medical treatments and supplies, creating a financial burden for those families.
3. Of the $327 billion, $90 billion is spent on research to prevent or cure diabetes.
4. The average patient spends or pays approximately $17,000 a year for their diabetes.
5. California's cost to treat diabetes is 40 billion dollars, because it has the largest diabetic population.
6. As of the publication of this book the most updated total cost of diabetes is now a staggering $413 billion just from 2017.

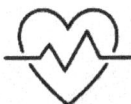

Additional Burdens of Diabetes

- The cost of diabetes also includes the patient's absence from work and other life events due to the need to visit the doctor and the time taken for treatments.
- In addition, some diabetics experience a reduction in sexual desire and productivity.
- There are also diseases/illnesses related to or caused by diabetic disabilities.
- There may be a reduction in the quality of life or premature death due to diabetes.
- Emergency room visits, doctor visits, hospital stays, outpatient visits, and medication costs can vary at each level of care.
- Other financial costs can include nursing home care, hospice care, and ambulance and medical transport costs.
- The cost to the patient will vary based on their medical insurance coverage.
- The cost of insulin in 1999 was $21.00 and rose to $332.00 by 2019, a 1481% increase. President Biden's 2022 Inflation Reduction Act caps the cost of insulin for Medicare patients at $35 per month.

The discoverers of insulin sold the patent for $1.00 in 1923 because they viewed it as unethical to profit from a lifesaving drug.

Step 13
Forbidden Topic

There is absolutely no need to be embarrassed when discussing intimate issues with your doctor. Sexual disorders can be a precursor to diabetes.

Sexual Disorders

1. As a diabetic, you may suffer from sexual disorders. These conditions may also cause psychological distress and decreased quality of life.
2. If you are male, erectile dysfunction (ED) could be the first sign of diabetes.
3. With ED, there is neurological and vascular impairment. In addition, the muscles of the penis may become smooth and relaxed.
4. Testosterone levels can be low due to diabetes. Blood tests can monitor this.

Normal sexual activity stimulates the release of nitric oxide at the cellular level in the penis. Nitric oxide is a vasodilator that expands blood vessels near the skin surface, leading to increased blood flow engorging the tissues of the penis, causing an erection.

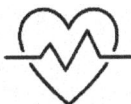

Sexual Disorder Treatments

- Medications such as Viagra or Cialis are vasodilators taken orally to produce an erection.
- Papaverine is an injectable that is injected directly into the erectile tissue of the penis.
- Additional treatments include a vacuum erection device or penile prosthesis.
- Other thoughts to consider are ejaculator dysfunctions that can cause infertility.

Women can also suffer from sexual disorders due to diabetes. Reduced interest in sex, sexual arousal, and possible orgasm disorder are a few. Just as Viagra improves blood flow for erection, it may also help women with a lowered libido to improve sexual arousal, achieve orgasm, and diminish the pain of dyspareunia.

Step 14
Other Effects of Diabetes

Diabetes can have an impact on lifestyle and longevity. It is essential to be aware of the complications that can arise from diabetes. Some of the more common effects of diabetes are as follows.

Dementia

1. Those with an early onset of DM (diabetes mellitus) and recurrent low blood glucose have a greater risk for the development of dementia.
2. Memory loss may occur from damage to the hippocampus, the memory center of the brain, as a result of diabetes.
3. Alzheimer's disease is linked to amyloid plaques which are found frequently in diabetics.

Depression

1. Controlling diabetes can be physically and emotionally exhausting. Staying on top of blood levels, injecting insulin, watching what you eat, etc., can be overwhelming and depressing.
2. Only about 35% of diabetics who have depression are diagnosed and treated.
3. Symptoms include loneliness, lack of interest, fatigue, and sleep disturbances.

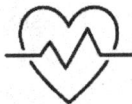

More Adverse Effects of Diabetes

Hearing Loss

Diabetics have twice the incidence of hearing loss due to direct injury to the sensory receptors in the inner ear from the thickening of the walls of small blood vessels.

Oral Diseases

- Dental cavities, tooth decay, gum disease, thrush, and dry mouth are commonly caused by diabetes.
- As a diabetic, you may experience a burning sensation in the mouth when blood sugar is not under control.
- Routine dental health care is a must. Always floss and brush your teeth and see your dentist twice a year.

Skin Disorders

- Dry skin, itching, recurrent infections, ulcerations (especially in the feet), and nail fungus are side effects of diabetes.
- Hair loss below the knees is another sign to be aware of.

Charcot's Joints

- Impairment walking due to nerve and vascular impairment causes muscle atrophy and deformity of the foot.
- To stop the progression of foot disease, see your primary care doctor or podiatrist.

Step 15
Live Life to the Fullest: Recommendations

A diagnosis of diabetes is not a death sentence. As a diabetic and a doctor, I have lived a good life for the past 32 years since being diagnosed.

1. Upon diagnosis take action! Be in control of your life. After all, it is your health and your responsibility.
2. To avoid complications, it is imperative to follow the advice of your physicians and nutritionists.
3. Practice portion control by eating more small meals during the day. This helps keep blood glucose under control rather than eating large portions in one sitting.
4. Some changes in your diet will be necessary. Avoid eating simple starches like potatoes and pasta, fried foods, fast foods, and sodas.

And always drink plenty of water!

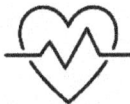

Other Recommendations

Monitoring your diet is likely the most important step you take in managing your diabetes.

- The Mediterranean diet is a very healthy lifestyle choice. It is also recommended to avoid Alzheimer's and inflammation.
- When it comes to grocery shopping, always look at the labels for sugar and fat content. Remember to shop the perimeter of the store where the fresh food is generally displayed; avoid the aisles.
- Moving and staying active is important. Regular exercise helps keep your weight and blood readings under control.
- Always take your prescribed medication as directed.
- Life is unpredictable. You never know from day to day what life will bring your way. With that said, try to avoid chronic and stressful situations whenever possible.

Finally, you only have one go-around in this life. So, live life to its fullest by adopting and following all the suggestions and advice in this guide to diabetes. To your good health!

You've Finished. Before you go…

Post/Share that you finished this book.

Please star rate this book.

Reviews are solid gold to writers. Please take a few minutes to give us some itty bitty feedback.

About the Author

Himmet Dajee, MD, FACS, was born in
Cape Town, South Africa. He completed
cardiothoracic surgery training at UCLA and
practiced for 25 years in both Los Angeles
and Orange County. Dr. Dajee is a board-
certified cardiothoracic surgeon. He is a
Fellow of the American College of Surgeons
and American College of Chest Physicians,
as well as a member of the Society of
Thoracic Surgeons.

To maintain a balanced life, Dr. Dajee loves
spending time with his wife and his two
wonderful daughters. He retired from active
practice in 2006 but didn't sit idle. He joined
a managed care health plan despite having
undergone two heart surgeries of his own.

He enjoys working daily providing health
care to the vulnerable population of Orange
County, California. In his spare time, Dr.
Dajee wrote his memoir titled, *A Boy Named
Courage: A Surgeon's Memoir of Apartheid*
(coauthored with Patrice Apodaca).

If you enjoyed this Itty Bitty™ Book you might also like…

- **Your Amazing Itty Bitty™ Alzheimer's Book** by Dung Trinh, MD

- **Your Amazing Itty Bitty™ Cancer Book** by Jacqueline Kreple

- **Your Amazing Itty Bitty™ Aging Well Book** by Michele McHenry

Or any of the other Amazing Itty Bitty™ books available online at www.IttyBittyPublishig.com

You've Been Diagnosed with Diabetes or Pre-Diabetes, Now What?

15 things you need to know to understand the power you have living with diabetes.

You can live a normal productive life with diabetes and very often it can be reversed. Diabetes is a worldwide epidemic, and most often life choices bring it on.

Poor food choices, stress, and lack of exercise are the main contributing factors that lead to Type 2 diabetes. You may have inherited genes or been infected by viruses that caused Type 1 diabetes; however, life choices can lessen the dangers associated with the disease. In this Itty Bitty™ book, Dr. Himmet Dajee discusses ways to reduce the effects of diabetes so it doesn't take over your body's internal organs. Diabetes is ranked as the seventh leading cause of death. You have the power to take charge and live the life you desire, but you must be proactive!

In this book you will learn:

- Appropriate treatments
- What the complications are
- Ways of prevention
- And so much more

If you are ready to reclaim your life and take charge of your diabetes pick up a copy of this informative Itty Bitty™ book today!